# SLIM & SATISTY

COOKBOOK

**DELICIOUS WEIGHT LOSS RECIPES**

# SUSAN L. SMITH

**Copyright © 2024 SUSAN L. SMITH**

All rights reserved. No part of this publication may be reproduced, distributed, or transmitted in any form or by any means, including photocopying, recording, or other electronic or mechanical methods, without the prior written permission of the publisher, except in the case of brief quotations embodied in critical reviews and certain other noncommercial uses permitted by copyright law.

# Table of Contents

Chapter 1 ............................................................. 7

  Breakfast support ............................................. 7

    1. Greek yogurt parfait with fruit and nuts ............ 7

    2. Avocado toast with a fried egg ........................... 8

    3. Omelet with spinach and feta ............................ 10

    4. Banana Oatmeal Pancakes .............................. 12

    5. Chia seed pudding ........................................... 13

Chapter 2 ............................................................ 15

  Light Lunches ................................................... 15

    1: Quinoa and vegetable salad ............................. 15

    2: Chicken and avocado wrap .............................. 17

    3: Lentil and spinach soup ................................... 19

    4: Turkey and vegetable stir-fry .......................... 20

    5: Chickpea and Avocado Salad .......................... 22

Chapter 3 ............................................................ 24

  Slim Suppers .................................................... 24

    1: Grilled chicken on lemon and herbs with quinoa vegetables ......................................................... 24

2: Baked salmon with asparagus and sweet potatoes...............................................................26

3: Turkey and vegetable stir-fry .......................28

4: Stuffed peppers wrapped in vegetables ............30

5: Spaghetti Squash with Turkey Marinara..........31

## Chapter 4...............................................................34

Smart Snacks ......................................................34

Why smart snacking matters?..............................34

Tips for smart snacks...........................................35

Smart snack recipes ................................................35

1. Greek yogurt with honey and almonds.............35

2. Vegetarian sticks with hummus......................36

3. Apple slices with peanut butter .......................37

4. Cottage cheese and pineapple........................38

5. Almond and berry parfait ...............................39

## Chapter 5...............................................................41

Guilt-Free Desserts ..................................................41

1: Chocolate Avocado Mousse...............................41

2: Baked apple slices with cinnamon ...................43

3: Greek Yogurt Berry Parfait...............................44

4: Banana Oatmeal Cookies ..................................45
5: Chia seed pudding ........................................47

## Chapter 6 ..............................................................48
### Meal Prep Magic ....................................................48
Tips for successful food preparation ..................48
Recipes........................................................................49
1: Chicken and vegetable stir-fry .......................49
2: Quinoa and Black Bean Salad........................51
3: Turkey meatballs with zucchini noodles..........53
4: Lentil and vegetable soup................................55
5: Greek Yogurt and Berry Parfaits.....................57

## Chapter 7 ..............................................................58
### Quick and Easy Recipes ........................................58
1: Chicken stir-fry with vegetables.....................58
2: Greek yogurt chicken salad .............................60
3: Vegetarian omelette..........................................62
4: Black Bean and Corn Salad.............................63
5: Zucchini noodles with pesto............................65

## Chapter 8 ..............................................................67
### Vegetarian and Vegan Options..............................67

1: Quinoa and peppers stuffed with black beans ..67
   2: Lentil and vegetable stir-fry ..............................69
   3: Sweet Potato and Chickpea Curry ...................70
   4: Spaghetti squash with tomatoes and basil ........72
   5: Black Bean and Avocado Salad .......................73
 Chapter 9 ....................................................................... 75
   Healthy Eating on a Budget.....................................75
   Tips for affordable healthy eating: .......................75
 Affordable and healthy recipes:................................76
   1. Black bean and corn salad ................................76
   2. Chicken and vegetable stir-fry..........................77
   3. Vegetable and lentil soup .................................79
   4. Baked Sweet Potatoes with Black Bean Salsa ..80
   5. Quinoa and peppers stuffed with vegetables ....82
 Chapter 10......................................................................84
   Smoothies and Drinks..............................................84
   1. Green Detox Smoothie ......................................84
   2. Berry Protein Smoothie ....................................85
   3. Tropical Paradise Smoothie..............................86
   4. Spicy citrus green tea........................................87

Tips for making the perfect smoothie ................... 89
Conclusion ................................................................ 91
Adopting a healthier lifestyle ................................ 91
Stay motivated and consistent ............................... 92
Additional resources ............................................... 92

# CHAPTER 1

## BREAKFAST SUPPORT

Breakfast is often touted as the most important meal of the day, and for good reason. A nutritious breakfast can jump-start your metabolism, fuel your morning activities, and set a positive tone for the rest of your day. In this chapter, we'll explore a number of delicious, low-calorie breakfast recipes that are satisfying and easy to make. Whether you're rushing out the door or enjoying a leisurely morning, these recipes will help you stick to your weight loss goals.

### 1. Greek yogurt parfait with fruit and nuts

Preparation time: 5 minutes

Servings: 1

*Ingredients:*

- 1 cup nonfat Greek yogurt
- 1/2 cup mixed fruit (strawberries, blueberries, raspberries)
- 1 spoon of honey

- 2 tablespoons of granola
- 1 tablespoon chopped almonds or walnuts

## *Instruction:*

- Yogurt layer: Pour half of the Greek yogurt into a glass or bowl.
- Add the berries: Add half of the mixed berries on top.
- Repeat the layers: Add the remaining yogurt, then the rest of the berries.
- Drizzle with honey: Drizzle honey over the top.
- Finish with Crunch: Top the parfait with granola and nuts.

## *Nutritional information (per serving):*

- Calories: 220
- Protein: 15 g
- Carbohydrates: 30 g
- Fat: 6g

## 2. Avocado toast with a fried egg

Preparation time: 10 minutes

Cooking time: 5 minutes

Servings: 1

***Ingredients:***

- 1 slice of whole wheat bread
- 1/2 ripe avocado
- 1 egg
- Salt and pepper to taste
- Optional: Red pepper flakes, fresh herbs or lemon juice

***Instruction:***

- Toast bread: Toast a slice of whole wheat bread until golden.
- Prepare the avocado: In a bowl, mash the avocado with a fork until smooth. Add salt and pepper to taste.
- To poach the eggs: Fill a saucepan with water and bring to a gentle boil. Crack the eggs into a small bowl, then carefully slide them into the boiling water. Cook for 3-4 minutes until the white is set but the yolk is still runny.
- Assembly: Spread mashed avocado on toasted bread. Place a fried egg on top.

- Garnish and serve: Add toppings if desired. Serve immediately.

***Nutritional information (per serving):***

- Calories: 250
- Protein: 12 g
- Carbohydrates: 20 g
- Fat: 15 g

## 3. Omelet with spinach and feta

Preparation time: 5 minutes

Cooking time: 10 minutes

Servings: 1

***Ingredients:***

- 2 large eggs
- 1/2 cup fresh spinach, chopped
- 1/4 cup feta cheese, crumbled
- 1 tablespoon milk (optional)
- Salt and pepper to taste
- 1 teaspoon of olive oil

## *Instruction:*

- Whisk the eggs: Whisk the eggs, milk (if using), salt and pepper in a bowl.
- Cook the spinach: Heat the olive oil in a nonstick skillet over medium heat. Add spinach and cook until wilted, about 2 minutes.
- Add the eggs: Pour the egg mixture over the spinach. Let it cook for about 2-3 minutes until the edges start to set.
- Add Feta: Sprinkle half of the omelette with feta cheese.
- To fold and finish: Fold the omelette in half and cook for another 1-2 minutes until the eggs are fully cooked. Serve hot.

## *Nutritional information (per serving):*

- Calories: 200
- Protein: 15 g
- Carbohydrates: 3 g
- Fat: 15 g

## 4. Banana Oatmeal Pancakes

Preparation time: 5 minutes

Cooking time: 10 minutes

Servings: 2

*Ingredients:*

- 1 ripe banana
- 1 cup rolled oats
- 2 large eggs
- 1/2 teaspoon baking powder
- 1/2 teaspoon cinnamon
- 1/4 cup milk (dairy or non-dairy)
- Optional: 1 teaspoon vanilla extract, fresh berries for topping

*Instruction:*

- Mix the ingredients: In a blender, combine the banana, oats, eggs, baking powder, cinnamon and milk. Blend until smooth.
- To cook the pancakes: Heat a non-stick frying pan over medium heat. Pour about 1/4 cup batter into the pan for each pancake. Cook for 2-3 minutes until bubbles form on the surface, then

flip and cook for another 1-2 minutes until golden.
- Serving: Serve the pancakes warm, topped with fresh fruit as desired.

***Nutritional information (per serving):***

- Calories: 270
- Protein: 10 g
- Carbohydrates: 45 g
- Fat: 6g

## 5. Chia seed pudding

Prep time: 5 minutes (plus chilling overnight)

Servings: 2

***Ingredients:***

- 1/4 cup chia seeds
- 1 cup unsweetened almond milk (or any milk)
- 1 tablespoon of honey or maple syrup
- 1/2 teaspoon of vanilla extract
- Optional toppings: Fresh fruit, nuts, granola

## *Instruction:*

- Mix the ingredients: In a bowl or glass, mix the chia seeds, almond milk, honey and vanilla extract.
- Refrigerate: Cover and refrigerate overnight or at least 4 hours until the mixture thickens to a custard-like consistency.
- To serve: Stir the puddings before serving. Top with fresh fruit, nuts or granola if you like.

## *Nutritional information (per serving):*

- Calories: 180
- Protein: 6 g
- Carbohydrates: 20 g
- Fat: 9g

# CHAPTER 2

## LIGHT LUNCHES

Lunch is an essential meal that will help you maintain your energy levels throughout the day. It should be balanced, nutritious and satisfying to avoid afternoon slumps and unhealthy snacking. In this chapter, we offer a variety of light lunch recipes that are not only delicious, but also in line with your weight loss goals. Each recipe includes a detailed list of ingredients, step-by-step instructions, preparation tips and serving suggestions to make your lunch enjoyable and beneficial to your weight loss journey.

**1: Quinoa and vegetable salad**

Preparation time: 15 minutes

Cooking time: 15 minutes

Servings: 2

*Ingredients:*

- 1 cup quinoa, rinsed
- 2 cups of water
- 1 cup cherry tomatoes, halved
- 1 cucumber, diced
- 1 red pepper, diced
- 1/4 cup red onion, finely chopped
- 1/4 cup fresh parsley, chopped
- 2 tablespoons of olive oil
- 2 tablespoons of lemon juice
- Salt and pepper to taste

*Instruction:*

- Cook the quinoa: In a medium saucepan, combine the quinoa and water. Bring to a boil, then reduce the heat to low, cover and simmer for about 15 minutes or until the water is absorbed. Prick with a fork and let cool.
- Prepare the vegetables: While the quinoa is cooking, chop the cherry tomatoes, cucumber, bell pepper, red onion and parsley.
- Mix the ingredients: In a large bowl, combine the cooked quinoa, chopped vegetables and parsley.

- Salad Dressing: In a small bowl, mix olive oil, lemon juice, salt and pepper. Pour over the quinoa mixture and toss to coat evenly.
- Serving: Divide the salad into two portions and serve immediately or refrigerate for later.

*Nutritional information (per serving):*

- Calories: 320
- Protein: 8 g
- Carbohydrates: 42 g
- Fat: 14g

## 2: Chicken and avocado wrap

Preparation time: 10 minutes

Cooking time: 10 minutes

Servings: 1

*Ingredients:*

- 1 whole wheat tortilla
- 1/2 avocado, sliced
- 1/2 cup cooked chicken breast, chopped
- 1/4 cup lettuce, chopped

- 1/4 cup tomatoes, diced
- 1 tablespoon of Greek yogurt
- 1 teaspoon lime juice
- Salt and pepper to taste

## *Instruction:*

- Prepare the ingredients: Cut the avocado, cut the chicken, cut the lettuce and dice the tomato.
- Make the dressing: In a small bowl, mix the Greek yogurt, lime juice, salt and pepper.
- To assemble the wrap: Lay the tortilla flat and spread the yogurt topping in the center. Add the avocado slices, chicken, lettuce and tomatoes.
- Wrap it up: Fold the sides of the tortilla over the filling, then roll up the bottom tightly to secure the wrap.
- To serve: If desired, cut in half and serve immediately.

## *Nutritional information (per serving):*

- Calories: 350
- Protein: 25 g
- Carbohydrates: 30 g
- Fat: 15 g

## 3: Lentil and spinach soup

Preparation time: 10 minutes

Cooking time: 30 minutes

Servings: 4

*Ingredients:*

- 1 cup dry lentils, rinsed
- 6 cups of vegetable broth
- 1 onion, chopped
- 2 carrots, chopped
- 2 celery stalks, chopped
- 3 cloves of garlic, chopped
- 1 teaspoon cumin
- 1/2 teaspoon turmeric
- 1/2 teaspoon paprika
- 4 cups fresh spinach
- Salt and pepper to taste

*Instruction:*

- Sauteed Vegetables: Heat a little oil in a large pot over medium heat. Add onion, carrot and celery. Fry for 5-7 minutes until the vegetables are soft.

- Add garlic and spices: Add garlic, cumin, turmeric and paprika. Cook for another 1-2 minutes until fragrant.
- Cook the lentils: Add the lentils and vegetable stock. Bring to the boil, then reduce the heat and simmer for 25-30 minutes until the lentils are tender.
- Add the spinach: Stir in the fresh spinach and cook for another 2-3 minutes until wilted.
- Season with salt and serve: Season with salt and pepper to taste. Serve hot.

*Nutritional information (per serving):*

- Calories: 180
- Protein: 12 g
- Carbohydrates: 30 g
- Fat: 2g

## 4: Turkey and vegetable stir-fry

Preparation time: 10 minutes

Cooking time: 15 minutes

Servings: 2

## *Ingredients:*

- 1/2 lb ground turkey
- 1 red pepper, sliced
- 1 zucchini, sliced
- 1 cup broccoli florets
- 2 cloves of garlic, chopped
- 1 tablespoon of soy sauce
- 1 tablespoon of olive oil
- 1 teaspoon of sesame oil
- Salt and pepper to taste

## *Instruction:*

- Cook the turkey: Heat the olive oil in a large skillet over medium-high heat. Add the ground turkey and cook until browned, breaking it up with a spoon, about 5-7 minutes.
- Add the vegetables: Add the peppers, zucchini and broccoli to the pan. Cook for another 5 minutes until the vegetables are tender.
- Add the garlic and soy sauce: Stir in the garlic, soy sauce, and sesame oil. Cook for another 1-2 minutes until well combined.

- Season with salt and serve: Season with salt and pepper to taste. Serve immediately.

*Nutritional information (per serving):*

- Calories: 270
- Protein: 28 g
- Carbohydrates: 12 g
- Fat: 12g

## 5: Chickpea and Avocado Salad

Preparation time: 10 minutes

Cooking time: None

Servings: 2

*Ingredients:*

- 1 can (15 ounces) chickpeas, drained and rinsed
- 1 avocado, diced
- 1/4 cup red onion, finely chopped
- 1/4 cup fresh cilantro, chopped
- 1 tablespoon of olive oil
- 1 tablespoon of lemon juice
- Salt and pepper to taste

*Instruction:*

- Prepare the ingredients: Dice the avocado and chop the red onion and cilantro.
- Mix the ingredients: In a large bowl, combine the chickpeas, avocado, red onion and cilantro.
- Salad dressing: Drizzle with olive oil and lemon juice. Stir gently to combine.
- Season with salt and serve: Season with salt and pepper to taste. Serve immediately.

*Nutritional information (per serving):*

- Calories: 320
- Protein: 10 g
- Carbohydrates: 32 g
- Fat: 18g

# CHAPTER 3

## SLIM SUPPERS

Dinner is often the most anticipated meal of the day, especially after a long day at work or activities. However, it can also be a challenging time for those trying to lose weight. The key to a satisfying and healthy dinner is to balance taste with nutrition to ensure your meal is filling and low in calories. In this chapter, you'll find a variety of hearty dinner recipes designed to help you maintain your weight loss goals without sacrificing taste.

### 1: Grilled chicken on lemon and herbs with quinoa vegetables

Preparation time: 15 minutes

Cooking time: 25 minutes

Servings: 4

*Ingredients:*

**For the chicken:**

- 4 boneless and skinless chicken breasts
- 1 lemon (juice and peel)
- 2 cloves of garlic, minced
- 2 tablespoons of olive oil
- 1 teaspoon of dried oregano
- 1 teaspoon of dried thyme
- Salt and pepper to taste

**For vegetarian quinoa:**

- 1 cup quinoa
- 2 cups of vegetable broth
- 1 bell pepper, diced
- 1 zucchini, diced
- 1 cup cherry tomatoes, halved
- 1/4 cup chopped fresh parsley
- 1 tablespoon of olive oil
- Salt and pepper to taste

*Instruction:*

- Marinate the chicken: In a bowl, combine the lemon juice and zest, garlic, olive oil, oregano,

thyme, salt and pepper. Add the chicken breasts and coat well. Marinate for at least 15 minutes.
- Cook with quinoa: Rinse the quinoa under cold water. Bring vegetable broth to a boil in a medium saucepan. Add the quinoa, reduce the heat to low, cover and cook for 15 minutes until the liquid is absorbed. Fluff with a fork.
- Prepare the vegetables: Heat the olive oil in a large skillet over medium heat. Add pepper and zucchini, sauté for 5 minutes. Add the cherry tomatoes and cook for another 2-3 minutes. Stir in the cooked quinoa and parsley. Season with salt and pepper.
- Grill the chicken: Preheat the grill or grill pan to medium-high heat. Grill the chicken for 6-7 minutes per side or until cooked through.
- To serve: Place grilled chicken on plates with vegetable quinoa.

## 2: Baked salmon with asparagus and sweet potatoes

Preparation time: 10 minutes

Cooking time: 25 minutes

Servings: 4

## *Ingredients:*

- 4 salmon fillets
- 1 bunch asparagus, chopped
- 2 large sweet potatoes, peeled and diced
- 2 tablespoons of olive oil
- 1 lemon (sliced)
- 1 teaspoon of garlic powder
- 1 teaspoon paprika
- Salt and pepper to taste

## *Instruction:*

- Preheat oven: Preheat oven to 400°F (200°C).
- Prepare the sweet potatoes: Place the sweet potatoes on a baking sheet, drizzle with 1 tablespoon of olive oil and season with salt, pepper, garlic powder and paprika. Stir to coat evenly.
- Bake the sweet potatoes: Bake for 10 minutes.
- Prepare the salmon and asparagus: While the sweet potatoes are baking, place the salmon fillets and asparagus on another baking sheet.

- Drizzle with the remaining olive oil, season with salt and pepper and place lemon slices.
- Bake everything together: After 10 minutes of baking the sweet potatoes, place the tray with the salmon and asparagus in the oven. Bake for an additional 15 minutes, or until the salmon is cooked through and flakes easily with a fork.
- Serve: Arrange the baked salmon, asparagus and sweet potatoes on plates and serve immediately.

### 3: Turkey and vegetable stir-fry

Preparation time: 15 minutes

Cooking time: 15 minutes

Servings: 4

*Ingredients:*

- 1 lb ground turkey
- 1 cup broccoli florets
- 1 bell pepper, sliced
- 1 carrot, thinly sliced
- 1 zucchini, sliced

- 2 cloves of garlic, minced
- 1 tablespoon fresh ginger, minced
- 2 tablespoons soy sauce (low sodium)
- 1 tablespoon hoisin sauce
- 1 tablespoon of olive oil
- 1 teaspoon of sesame oil
- 2 green onions, sliced
- 1 tablespoon sesame seeds (optional)

### *Instruction:*

- Prepare the sauce: In a small bowl, combine the soy sauce, hoisin sauce, and sesame oil. Set aside.
- Cook the turkey: In a large skillet or wok, heat the olive oil over medium-high heat. Add ground turkey and cook until browned, about 5-7 minutes. Remove from pan and set aside.
- Sauté the vegetables: In the same pan, add the garlic and ginger. Fry for 1 minute. Add the broccoli, peppers, carrots and zucchini. Cook for 5-7 minutes until the vegetables are tender.
- Combine and Season: Return the cooked turkey to the pan. Pour in the sauce and toss to

combine. Cook for another 2-3 minutes until heated through.
- Serve: Garnish with green onions and sesame seeds. Serve hot.

## 4: Stuffed peppers wrapped in vegetables

Preparation time: 15 minutes

Cooking time: 40 minutes

Servings: 4

### *Ingredients:*

- 4 large peppers, cut off the tops and remove the seeds
- 1 cup cooked brown rice
- 1 can of black beans, drained and rinsed
- 1 cup corn kernels (fresh or frozen)
- 1 cup chopped tomatoes
- 1 small onion, finely chopped
- 2 cloves of garlic, minced
- 1 teaspoon cumin
- 1 teaspoon chili powder

- 1 tablespoon of olive oil
- Salt and pepper to taste
- 1/2 cup grated cheddar cheese (optional)
- Fresh cilantro for garnish

## *Instruction:*

- Preheat oven: Preheat oven to 375°F (190°C).
- Prepare the filling: Heat the olive oil in a large skillet over medium heat. Add onion and garlic, sauté for 3 minutes. Add the black beans, corn, diced tomatoes, cooked brown rice, cumin, chili powder, salt and pepper. Cook for another 5 minutes until heated through.
- Stuff the peppers: Spoon the filling into each pepper and gently roll it up. Place the stuffed peppers in a baking dish.
- Bake: Cover the bowl with foil and bake for 30 minutes. If using cheese, remove the foil, sprinkle with cheese and bake uncovered for a further 10 minutes until the cheese has melted.
- Serve: Garnish with fresh cilantro and serve hot.

## 5: Spaghetti Squash with Turkey Marinara

Preparation time: 15 minutes

Cooking time: 45 minutes

Servings: 4

## *Ingredients:*

- 1 large spaghetti squash
- 1 lb ground turkey
- 1 can crushed tomatoes (28 oz)
- 1 small onion, finely chopped
- 3 cloves of garlic, chopped
- 1 teaspoon dried basil
- 1 teaspoon of dried oregano
- 1 tablespoon of olive oil
- Salt and pepper to taste
- Fresh basil for garnish (optional)
- Grated Parmesan (optional)

## *Instruction:*

- Preheat oven: Preheat oven to 400°F (200°C).
- Prepare the pumpkin: Cut the spaghetti squash in half lengthwise and scoop out the seeds. Drizzle with olive oil and season with salt and pepper.

Place cut side down on baking sheet and bake for 40 minutes or until tender.
- Cook the turkey: Heat the olive oil in a large skillet over medium heat. Add onion and garlic, sauté for 3 minutes. Add ground turkey and cook until browned, about 5-7 minutes.
- Prepare Marinara: Stir in crushed tomatoes, dried basil and oregano. Season with salt and pepper. Cook for 15-20 minutes, stirring occasionally.
- Prepare the squash: Once the squash is cooked, use a fork to scrape the squash strands into a large bowl.
- Serve: Divide spaghetti squash among plates and fill with turkey marinara. Garnish with fresh basil and grated parmesan to taste.

# CHAPTER 4
## SMART SNACKS

Snacking can be an essential part of a balanced diet, especially when you're trying to lose weight. The key to success is choosing snacks that are satisfying and nutritious. In this chapter, we'll explore different smart snack options to help you stay full, energized, and on track to your weight loss goals.

### Why smart snacking matters?

Choosing the right snack can help you:

Control hunger: Avoid overeating at meals by keeping your hunger at bay.

Boost energy: Maintain steady energy levels throughout the day.

Metabolism Support: Keep your metabolism active and prevent it from slowing down.

### Tips for smart snacks

Portion control: Portion snacks ahead of time to avoid overeating.

Balance: Combine protein, healthy fats and fiber for sustained satiety.

Timing: Space out snacks between meals to keep your blood sugar stable.

## SMART SNACK RECIPES

### 1. Greek yogurt with honey and almonds

Preparation time: 5 minutes

Servings: 1

*Ingredients:*

- 1 cup plain Greek yogurt
- 1 spoon of honey
- 10 almonds, chopped
- Optional: sprinkle with cinnamon or fresh fruit

*Instruction:*

- Mix the ingredients: In a bowl, mix the Greek yogurt and honey until well combined.
- Top with almonds: Sprinkle chopped almonds on top.
- Optional extras: Add a pinch of cinnamon or fresh fruit for extra flavor and nutrients.
- Serving: Enjoy immediately as a delicious protein-packed snack.

*Nutritional information (per serving):*

- Calories: 200
- Protein: 15 g
- Carbohydrates: 18 g
- Fat: 8g


## 2. Vegetarian sticks with hummus

Preparation time: 10 minutes

Servings: 2

*Ingredients:*

- 1 cup baby carrots

- 1 cup of cucumber sticks
- 1 cup bell pepper strips
- 1/2 cup hummus

*Instruction:*

- Preparing the vegetables: Wash the vegetables and cut them into strips or noodles.
- Serve with hummus: Place the veggie sticks on a plate and serve with hummus.
- Serving: This snack can be stored in an airtight container for up to 2 days.

*Nutritional information (per serving):*

- Calories: 150
- Protein: 4 g
- Carbohydrates: 20 g
- Fat: 7g

### 3. Apple slices with peanut butter

Preparation time: 5 minutes

Servings: 1

*Ingredients:*

- 1 medium apple
- 1 tablespoon natural peanut butter

*Instruction:*

- Cut the apple: Remove the core from the apple and cut it into thin slices.
- Spread with peanut butter: Spread a thin layer of peanut butter on each apple slice.
- Serving: Enjoy immediately. This snack is great for on the go.

*Nutritional information (per serving):*

- Calories: 180
- Protein: 3 g
- Carbohydrates: 25 g
- Fat: 8g

### 4. Cottage cheese and pineapple

Preparation time: 5 minutes

Servings: 1

*Ingredients:*

- 1/2 cup low-fat cottage cheese
- 1/2 cup pineapple chunks (fresh or canned in juice, drained)

*Instruction:*

- Combine the ingredients: In a small bowl, combine the cottage cheese and pineapple chunks.
- Serve: Enjoy immediately or refrigerate for later.
- Serving: Perfect as a quick and refreshing snack.

*Nutritional information (per serving):*

- Calories: 120
- Protein: 10 g
- Carbohydrates: 15 g
- Fat: 2g

## 5. Almond and berry parfait

Preparation time: 5 minutes

Servings: 1

## *Ingredients:*

- 1/2 cup mixed fruit (strawberries, blueberries, raspberries)
- 1/2 cup low-fat Greek yogurt
- 2 tablespoons chopped almonds
- 1 teaspoon of honey

## *Instruction:*

- Layer ingredients: Layer Greek yogurt, mixed berries and sliced almonds in a glass or bowl.
- Drizzle with honey: For added sweetness, drizzle with honey.
- Serve: Enjoy immediately.
- Serving: This snack can be made in advance and refrigerated for up to 1 day.

## *Nutritional information (per serving):*

- Calories: 200
- Protein: 10 g
- Carbohydrates: 25 g
- Fat: 7g

# CHAPTER 5

## GUILT-FREE DESSERTS

Who says you can't have dessert while losing weight? The key is to choose desserts that satisfy your sweet tooth without derailing your progress. This chapter is dedicated to delicious, guilt-free desserts that are low in calories but high in flavor. Each recipe is designed to provide a healthier alternative to traditional desserts, allowing you to indulge guilt-free. Whether you're craving chocolate, fruit or something creamy, we've got something good for you.

### 1: Chocolate Avocado Mousse

*Ingredients:*

- 2 ripe avocados
- 1/4 cup unsweetened cocoa powder
- 1/4 cup honey or maple syrup
- 1/4 cup almond milk (unsweetened)

- 1 teaspoon of vanilla extract
- Pinch of salt
- Fresh berries or mint leaves for garnish (optional)

## *Instruction:*

- Preparing the avocado: Cut the avocado in half, remove the pit and scoop the pulp into a blender or food processor.
- Mix: Add cocoa powder, honey or maple syrup, almond milk, vanilla extract and a pinch of salt to a blender.
- Blend: Blend until mixture is smooth and creamy, stopping to scrape down sides as needed.
- Refrigerate: Transfer the mousse to serving bowls and refrigerate for at least 30 minutes to set.
- Serve: Before serving, garnish with fresh fruit or mint leaves as desired.

## *Nutritional information (per serving, makes 4 servings):*

- Calories: 200

- Protein: 3 g
- Carbohydrates: 26 g
- Fat: 12g

## 2: Baked apple slices with cinnamon

*Ingredients:*

- 4 large apples (any variety)
- 2 teaspoons of ground cinnamon
- 1 tablespoon coconut oil (melted)
- 2 tablespoons maple syrup or honey
- 1/4 cup chopped nuts (optional)

*Instruction:*

- Preheat oven: Preheat oven to 350°F (175°C).
- Prepare the apples: Remove the core from the apples and cut them into thin wedges.
- Mix the ingredients: In a large bowl, toss the apple slices with the melted coconut oil, cinnamon, and maple syrup or honey until evenly coated.

- Bake: Spread the apple slices in one layer on a baking sheet lined with baking paper. Sprinkle with chopped nuts, if using.
- Cooking: Bake for 20-25 minutes, or until the apples are soft and lightly caramelized.
- Serve: Serve warm as a stand-alone dessert or with a dollop of Greek yogurt.

*Nutritional information (per serving, makes 4 servings):*

- Calories: 150
- Protein: 1 g
- Carbohydrates: 26 g
- Fat: 5g

## 3: Greek Yogurt Berry Parfait

*Ingredients:*

- 2 cups plain Greek yogurt (non-fat or low-fat)
- 1 cup mixed fruit (blueberries, strawberries, raspberries)
- 2 spoons of honey
- 1/4 cup granola (optional)

- mint leaves for garnish (optional)

***Instruction:***

- Prepare the ingredients: If necessary, wash and chop the berries.
- Layer parfait: In a glass or bowl, layer 1/2 cup Greek yogurt, then a handful of mixed berries and drizzle with honey.
- Repeat: Repeat layers until yogurt and berries are used up.
- Top: If desired, sprinkle with granola and garnish with mint leaves.
- Serve: Serve immediately or refrigerate for up to an hour.

***Nutritional information (per serving, makes 4 servings):***

- Calories: 180
- Protein: 10 g
- Carbohydrates: 26 g
- Fat: 3g

## 4: Banana Oatmeal Cookies

## *Ingredients:*

- 2 ripe bananas
- 1 cup rolled oats
- 1/2 teaspoon of vanilla extract
- 1/4 cup dark chocolate chips (optional)
- 1/4 cup chopped nuts (optional)

## *Instruction:*

- Preheat the oven: Preheat the oven to 350°F (175°C) and line a baking sheet with parchment paper.
- Mash the bananas: In a large bowl, mash the bananas until smooth.
- Mix Ingredients: Stir in rolled oats and vanilla extract. Add chocolate chips and nuts, if using.
- Form the cookies: Pour the mixture by spoonfuls onto the prepared baking sheet and flatten them slightly with the back of a spoon.
- Bake: Bake for 15-20 minutes or until the cookies are golden brown.
- Cool: Leave to cool on a wire rack before serving.

*Nutritional information (per serving, makes 12 cookies):*

- Calories: 90
- Protein: 2 g
- Carbohydrates: 18 g
- Fat: 2g

### 5: Chia seed pudding

*Ingredients:*

- 1/4 cup chia seeds
- 1 cup almond milk (unsweetened)
- 1 tablespoon of honey or maple syrup
- 1/2 teaspoon of vanilla extract
- Fresh fruit or nuts for topping (optional)

*Instruction:*

- Combine the ingredients: In a medium bowl, whisk together the chia seeds, almond milk, honey or maple syrup, and vanilla extract.
- Refrigerate: Cover and refrigerate for at least 4 hours or overnight, until mixture thickens to a custard-like consistency.

- Mixing: Before serving, mix the puddings to break up any lumps.
- Serve: Spoon into serving bowls and top with fresh fruit or nuts, if desired.

*Nutritional information (per serving, makes 4 servings):*

- Calories: 150
- Protein: 4 g
- Carbohydrates: 15 g
- Fat: 8g

# CHAPTER 6
## MEAL PREP MAGIC

Meal prep is a game changer when it comes to maintaining a healthy diet and sticking to your weight loss goals. By taking a little time each week to plan and prepare your meals, you can save time, reduce stress and ensure you always have nutritious options on hand. This chapter takes you through the basics of meal preparation and gives you five tasty and practical recipes to get you started.

**Tips for successful food preparation**

1. Plan ahead: Choose recipes that are easy to prepare and store well. Make a shopping list to make sure you have all the ingredients you need.

2. Invest in quality containers: Use airtight containers to keep your food fresh. Glass containers are great for reheating, while BPA-free plastic containers are lightweight and portable.

3. Batch Cooking: Cook large batches of your favorite recipes and divide them into individual portions. That way, you'll have ready-to-eat meals throughout the week.

4. Balance your meals: Make sure each meal contains a good balance of protein, healthy fats and complex carbohydrates. This will keep you satisfied and energized.

5. Marking and date: Always mark containers with the name of the dish and the date of its preparation. This will help you keep track of what needs to be eaten first.

# RECIPES

### 1: Chicken and vegetable stir-fry

Preparation time: 15 minutes

Cooking time: 20 minutes

Servings: 4

*Ingredients:*

- 2 boneless skinless chicken breasts, cut into thin strips
- 2 tablespoons of olive oil
- 1 bell pepper, sliced
- 1 head of broccoli, cut into florets
- 2 carrots, sliced
- 1 onion, chopped
- 3 cloves of garlic, chopped
- 1/4 cup low-sodium soy sauce
- 2 spoons of honey

- 1 tablespoon of cornstarch
- 1/4 cup water
- Salt and pepper to taste

## *Instruction:*

- Make the sauce: In a small bowl, combine the soy sauce, honey, cornstarch, and water. Set aside.
- Cook the chicken: Heat 1 tablespoon olive oil in a large skillet over medium-high heat. Add the chicken noodles, season with salt and pepper, and cook until browned and cooked through, about 5-7 minutes. Remove the chicken from the pan and set aside.
- Fry the vegetables: In the same pan, add the remaining tablespoon of olive oil. Add the onion and garlic and cook for 2 minutes until fragrant. Add the peppers, broccoli and carrots and stir-fry for 5-7 minutes until golden.
- Combine and cook: Return the chicken to the pan and pour the sauce over the mixture. Mix well and let it boil for 2-3 minutes until the sauce thickens.

- Cool and store: Allow the stir-fry to cool before portioning into containers. Store in the fridge for up to 4 days.
- Serving: As a complete meal, serve with brown rice or quinoa.

## 2: Quinoa and Black Bean Salad

Preparation time: 15 minutes

Cooking time: 15 minutes

Servings: 4

### *Ingredients:*

- 1 cup quinoa
- 2 cups of water
- 1 can of black beans, drained and rinsed
- 1 cup cherry tomatoes, halved
- 1 red pepper, diced
- 1/4 cup red onion, finely chopped
- 1 avocado, diced
- 1/4 cup fresh cilantro, chopped
- Juice of 1 lime

- 2 tablespoons of olive oil
- Salt and pepper to taste

## *Instruction:*

- Cook the quinoa: Rinse the quinoa under cold water. Bring water to a boil in a medium saucepan. Add the quinoa, reduce to a simmer, cover and cook for 15 minutes until the water is absorbed. Prick with a fork and let cool.
- Combine the ingredients: In a large bowl, combine the cooked quinoa, black beans, cherry tomatoes, bell pepper, red onion, avocado, and cilantro.
- Salad Dressing: In a small bowl, combine lime juice, olive oil, salt and pepper. Pour over salad and toss to coat.
- Refrigerate and store: Divide the salad into containers. Store in the fridge for up to 4 days.
- Serving: Enjoy as a main dish or as a side dish with grilled chicken or fish.

## 3: Turkey meatballs with zucchini noodles

Preparation time: 20 minutes

Cooking time: 25 minutes

Servings: 4

## *Ingredients:*

- 1 pound ground turkey
- 1/4 cup breadcrumbs
- 1/4 cup grated Parmesan
- 1 egg
- 2 cloves of garlic, chopped
- 1 teaspoon of Italian seasoning
- Salt and pepper to taste
- 2 tablespoons of olive oil
- 4 medium courgettes, spiral
- 1 cup marinara sauce (about 2 cups)

## *Instruction:*

- Make the meatballs: In a large bowl, combine the ground turkey, breadcrumbs, Parmesan cheese, egg, garlic, Italian seasoning, salt and pepper. Stir until well combined to form small meatballs.

- Cook the meatballs: Heat 1 tablespoon olive oil in a large skillet over medium heat. Add the meatballs and cook until browned on all sides and cooked through, about 10-12 minutes. Remove from pan and set aside.
- Cook the zucchini noodles: In the same pan, add the remaining tablespoon of olive oil. Add the spiralized zucchini and cook for 3-4 minutes until softened.
- Combine and cook: Return the meatballs to the pan and pour the marinara sauce over them. Let it cook for 5 minutes until heated through.
- Refrigerate and store: Allow the bowl to cool before portioning into containers. Store in the fridge for up to 4 days.
- Serving: Serve as is or sprinkled with fresh basil and extra Parmesan.

## 4: Lentil and vegetable soup

Preparation time: 15 minutes

Cooking time: 45 minutes

Servings: 4

## *Ingredients:*

- 1 tablespoon of olive oil
- 1 onion, diced
- 2 cloves of garlic, chopped
- 2 carrots, diced
- 2 stalks of celery, diced
- 1 zucchini, diced
- 1 cup dried lentils, rinsed
- 1 can (14.5 oz) diced tomatoes
- 4 cups of vegetable broth
- 1 teaspoon of dried thyme
- 1 bay leaf
- Salt and pepper to taste
- Fresh parsley, chopped, for garnish

## *Instruction:*

- Saute the vegetables: Heat the olive oil in a large pot over medium heat. Add the onion and garlic and cook until softened, about 5 minutes. Add the carrot, celery and zucchini and cook for another 5 minutes.

- Add lentils and stock: Add lentils, diced tomatoes, vegetable stock, thyme, bay leaf, salt and pepper. Bring to a boil, then reduce the heat and simmer for 30-35 minutes, until the lentils are tender.
- Remove the bay leaf: Discard the bay leaf before serving.
- Cool and store: Allow soup to cool before portioning into containers. Store in the fridge for up to 5 days or freeze for up to 3 months.
- Serving: Garnish with fresh parsley and enjoy with a slice of whole wheat bread.

## **5: Greek Yogurt and Berry Parfaits**

Preparation time: 10 minutes

Servings: 4

*Ingredients:*

- 2 cups Greek yogurt

- 1 cup mixed fruit (blueberries, strawberries, raspberries)
- 1/2 cup granola
- 2 spoons of honey
- 1 teaspoon of vanilla extract

***Instruction:***

- Make the yogurt: In a medium bowl, mix the Greek yogurt with the honey and vanilla extract.
- To layer the parfaits: In four small containers or glasses, layer the yogurt, berries and granola. Start with a layer of yogurt, followed by berries and then granola. Repeat the layers until the containers are full.
- Refrigerate and store: Cover and refrigerate parfaits for up to 3 days.
- Dosage: Enjoy as a quick breakfast or a healthy snack.

# CHAPTER 7
## QUICK AND EASY RECIPES

In today's busy world, it can be difficult to find time to cook healthy meals. That's why this chapter is dedicated to quick and easy recipes that are great for busy days. These meals are not only easy to prepare, but they are also packed with nutrients to support your weight loss journey. Whether you're rushing to work in the morning, need a quick lunch between meetings, or want a hassle-free dinner after a long day, these recipes will help.

### 1: Chicken stir-fry with vegetables

Preparation time: 10 minutes

Cooking time: 15 minutes

Servings: 4

*Ingredients:*

- 2 boneless skinless chicken breasts, cut into thin strips
- 1 red pepper, sliced
- 1 yellow bell pepper, sliced
- 1 cup broccoli florets
- 1 cup split peas
- 1 medium carrot, julienned
- 2 cloves of garlic, minced
- 2 tablespoons soy sauce (low sodium)
- 1 tablespoon of olive oil
- 1 teaspoon of sesame oil
- 1 teaspoon cornstarch mixed with 1/4 cup water
- Cooked brown rice or quinoa (optional)

## *Instruction:*

- Heat the oils: In a large skillet or wok, heat the olive oil and sesame oil over medium-high heat.
- To cook the chicken: Add the chicken noodles and cook until they are pink, about 5-7 minutes. Remove the chicken from the pan and set aside.
- Cook the vegetables: In the same pan, add the garlic and cook for 30 seconds until fragrant. Add peppers, broccoli, peas and carrots. Fry for

- 5-7 minutes, stirring constantly, until the vegetables are soft.
- Combine the ingredients: Return the chicken to the pan. Add soy sauce and cornstarch mixture. Mix well and cook for another 2-3 minutes until the sauce thickens and coats the chicken and vegetables.
- Serving: Serve fried with cooked brown rice or quinoa, if desired.

*Nutritional information (per serving):*

- Calories: 250
- Protein: 26 g
- Carbohydrates: 15 g
- Fat: 10 g

## 2: Greek yogurt chicken salad

Preparation time: 10 minutes

Cooking time: 0 minutes (use precooked chicken)

Servings: 2

*Ingredients:*

- 1 cup cooked chicken breast, cut into pieces
- 1/2 cup Greek yogurt
- 1/4 cup diced celery
- 1/4 cup chopped red onion
- 1/4 cup halved grapes
- 1 tablespoon chopped fresh dill
- 1 tablespoon of lemon juice
- Salt and pepper to taste
- Lettuce leaves or whole wheat bread to serve

## *Instruction:*

- Mix the ingredients: In a large bowl, combine the chopped chicken, Greek yogurt, celery, red onion, grapes, dill and lemon juice.
- Spices: Salt and pepper to taste. Mix until well combined.
- Serve: Serve the chicken salad on lettuce leaves as a low-carb option or as a sandwich filling with whole wheat bread.

## *Nutritional information (per serving):*

- Calories: 200
- Protein: 25 g
- Carbohydrates: 10 g

- Fat: 7g

## 3: Vegetarian omelette

Preparation time: 5 minutes

Cooking time: 10 minutes

Servings: 1

***Ingredients:***

- 2 large eggs
- 1/4 cup chopped tomatoes
- 1/4 cup chopped paprika
- 1/4 cup spinach leaves, chopped
- 1/4 cup chopped mushrooms
- 1 tablespoon milk (optional)
- Salt and pepper to taste
- 1 teaspoon of olive oil

***Instruction:***

- To prepare the eggs: In a bowl, beat the eggs with the milk (if using), salt and pepper.
- Cook the vegetables: Heat the olive oil in a non-stick pan over medium heat. Add the tomatoes,

- peppers, spinach and mushrooms. Cook for 3-4 minutes until the vegetables are tender.
- Cook the omelette: Pour the eggs over the vegetables in the pan. Cook for 2-3 minutes until edges begin to set. Carefully turn the omelette over and cook for another 2 minutes until completely set.
- Serve: Serve immediately with a side of whole wheat toast or a small salad.

## *Nutritional information (per serving):*

- Calories: 200
- Protein: 14 g
- Carbohydrates: 6 g
- Fat: 14g

## **4: Black Bean and Corn Salad**

Preparation time: 10 minutes

Cooking time: 0 minutes

Servings: 4

## *Ingredients:*

- 1 can (15 ounces) black beans, rinsed and drained
- 1 cup corn kernels (fresh, frozen, or canned)
- 1 red pepper, diced
- 1/4 cup red onion, finely chopped
- 1/4 cup chopped fresh cilantro
- 2 tablespoons lime juice
- 1 tablespoon of olive oil
- Salt and pepper to taste

## *Instruction:*

- Combine the ingredients: In a large bowl, combine the black beans, corn, bell pepper, red onion, and cilantro.
- Dressing salad: In a small bowl, mix lime juice, olive oil, salt and pepper. Pour over bean mixture and toss to coat.
- Serve: Serve immediately or refrigerate for an hour to allow the flavors to meld.

## *Nutritional information (per serving):*

- Calories: 150
- Protein: 5 g
- Carbohydrates: 24 g

- Fat: 4g

## 5: Zucchini noodles with pesto

Preparation time: 10 minutes

Cooking time: 5 minutes

Servings: 2

*Ingredients:*

- 2 medium courgettes, spiraled into noodles
- 1/2 cup cherry tomatoes, halved
- 1/4 cup prepared pesto (store-bought or homemade)
- 1 tablespoon of olive oil
- 1/4 cup grated Parmesan cheese (optional)
- Salt and pepper to taste

*Instruction:*

- To cook the zucchini noodles: Heat the olive oil in a large skillet over medium heat. Add the zucchini noodles and cook for 2-3 minutes until tender.

- Add the pesto: Remove from the heat and toss the pasta with the pesto until evenly coated.
- Add the tomatoes: Add the cherry tomatoes and mix gently.
- Serve: Divide between two plates, sprinkle with Parmesan cheese if desired, and season with salt and pepper to taste.

*Nutritional information (per serving):*

- Calories: 200
- Protein: 6 g
- Carbohydrates: 10 g
- Fat: 16 g

# CHAPTER 8
## VEGETARIAN AND VEGAN OPTIONS

Switching to a plant-based diet can be a powerful tool for weight loss. Not only are vegetarian and vegan foods often lower in calories, they are also rich in nutrients, fibre and antioxidants that can improve overall health. This chapter is dedicated to providing you with delicious, satisfying plant-based recipes that are easy to prepare and perfect for supporting your weight loss goals.

### 1: Quinoa and peppers stuffed with black beans

Preparation time: 15 minutes

Cooking time: 40 minutes

Servings: 4

*Ingredients:*

- 4 large peppers

- 1 cup quinoa, rinsed
- 1 can (15 ounces) black beans, drained and rinsed
- 1 cup corn kernels (fresh or frozen)
- 1 can (14.5 oz) diced tomatoes
- 1 teaspoon cumin
- 1 teaspoon chili powder
- Salt and pepper to taste
- 1 cup grated vegan cheese (optional)
- Fresh cilantro for garnish

## *Instruction:*

- Preheat oven to 375°F (190°C). Cut the tops off the peppers and remove the seeds and membranes.
- In a medium saucepan, cook quinoa according to package directions.
- In a large bowl, combine the cooked quinoa, black beans, corn, diced tomatoes, cumin, chili powder, salt, and pepper.
- Stuff the peppers with the quinoa mixture and place them in a baking dish.
- Top stuffed peppers with grated vegan cheese, if using.

- Cover the dish with foil and bake for 30 minutes. Remove the foil and bake for another 10 minutes until the peppers are soft.
- Garnish with fresh cilantro before serving.

## 2: Lentil and vegetable stir-fry

Preparation time: 10 minutes

Cooking time: 20 minutes

Servings: 4

### *Ingredients:*

- 1 cup dried lentils, rinsed and drained
- 2 cups of vegetable broth
- 2 tablespoons of olive oil
- 1 red pepper, sliced
- 1 yellow bell pepper, sliced
- 1 zucchini, sliced
- 1 cup broccoli florets
- 2 cloves of garlic, minced
- 2 tablespoons soy sauce or tamari
- 1 teaspoon grated ginger

- 1 tablespoon of sesame seeds
- Fresh basil or cilantro for garnish

***Instruction:***

- Combine lentils and vegetable stock in a medium saucepan. Bring to a boil, then reduce the heat and simmer for about 20 minutes, until the lentils are tender. Drain the excess liquid.
- In a large skillet, heat the olive oil over medium-high heat. Add the garlic and ginger and sauté for 1 minute.
- Add peppers, zucchini and broccoli to the pan. Fry for 5-7 minutes, stirring constantly, until the vegetables are soft.
- Add the cooked lentils, soy sauce and sesame seeds to the pan. Stir to combine and reheat.
- Garnish with fresh basil or cilantro before serving.

### 3: Sweet Potato and Chickpea Curry

Preparation time: 10 minutes

Cooking time: 25 minutes

Servings: 4

## *Ingredients:*

- 1 tablespoon of coconut oil
- 1 onion, chopped
- 2 cloves of garlic, minced
- 1 tablespoon of grated ginger
- 1 tablespoon curry
- 1 teaspoon ground cumin
- 1 teaspoon of turmeric
- 1 can (14 ounces) coconut milk
- 2 large sweet potatoes, peeled and diced
- 1 can (15 ounces) chickpeas, drained and rinsed
- 1 cup of vegetable broth
- Salt and pepper to taste
- Fresh cilantro for garnish

## *Instruction:*

- In a large saucepan, heat the coconut oil over medium heat. Add the onion, garlic and ginger and sauté for 3-4 minutes until softened.
- Stir in the curry, cumin and turmeric and cook for 1 minute until fragrant.

- Add the sweet potatoes, chickpeas, coconut milk and vegetable broth. Bring to a boil, then reduce the heat and simmer for 20-25 minutes, until the sweet potatoes are tender.
- Season with salt and pepper to taste.
- Garnish with fresh cilantro before serving.

## 4: Spaghetti squash with tomatoes and basil

Preparation time: 10 minutes

Cooking time: 40 minutes

Servings: 4

### *Ingredients:*

- 1 large spaghetti squash
- 2 tablespoons of olive oil
- 2 cloves of garlic, minced
- 1 can (14.5 oz) diced tomatoes
- 1/4 cup fresh basil, chopped
- Salt and pepper to taste
- 1/4 cup vegan parmesan cheese (optional)

### *Instruction:*

- Preheat oven to 400°F (200°C). Cut the spaghetti squash in half lengthwise and remove the seeds.
- Place the squash halves cut side down on a baking sheet and bake for 30-40 minutes until tender.
- While the squash is baking, heat the olive oil in a large skillet over medium heat. Add the garlic and sauté for 1 minute.
- Add the chopped tomatoes and cook for 5-7 minutes until the sauce thickens slightly. Stir in fresh basil and season with salt and pepper.
- When the pumpkin is done, use a fork to scrape the flesh into spaghetti-like strands.
- Toss the spaghetti squash with the tomato sauce and sprinkle with vegan parmesan cheese if desired.

## 5: Black Bean and Avocado Salad

Preparation time: 10 minutes

Cooking time: None

Servings: 4

***Ingredients:***

- 2 cans (15 oz each) black beans, drained and rinsed
- 1 avocado, diced
- 1 red pepper, diced
- 1 small red onion, finely chopped
- 1 cup cherry tomatoes, halved
- 1/4 cup fresh cilantro, chopped
- 2 tablespoons of olive oil
- 2 tablespoons lime juice
- Salt and pepper to taste

***Instruction:***

- In a large bowl, combine the black beans, avocado, red pepper, red onion, cherry tomatoes and cilantro.
- In a small bowl, mix olive oil, lime juice, salt and pepper.
- Pour the dressing over the salad and toss to combine.
- Serve immediately or refrigerate for 2 hours to allow the flavors to meld.

- These recipes are designed to be not only healthy and low in calories, but also satisfying and delicious, making it easier for you to stick to your weight loss journey. Enjoy these plant-based foods and feel great about the positive effects they have on your health and well-being.

# CHAPTER 9

## HEALTHY EATING ON A BUDGET

Eating healthy doesn't have to make money. With a little planning and smart shopping, you can enjoy nutritious, delicious meals that support your weight loss goals without breaking the bank. This chapter guides you through budget shopping tips and gives you five affordable and healthy recipes.

**Tips for affordable healthy eating:**

- Plan your meals: Make a weekly meal plan and create a shopping list to avoid impulse purchases.
- Buy in bulk: Buy staples like grains, beans, and frozen vegetables in bulk to save money.
- Seasonal produce: Choose seasonal fruits and vegetables for better prices and freshness.
- Generic brands: Opt for store brands, which are often cheaper than name brands but just as good quality.
- Cook at home: Preparing meals at home is usually cheaper and healthier than eating out.
- Use leftovers: Incorporate leftovers into new meals to reduce waste and save money.

## AFFORDABLE AND HEALTHY RECIPES:

### 1. Black bean and corn salad

Preparation time: 10 minutes

Servings: 4

*Ingredients:*

- 1 can of black beans, drained and rinsed
- 1 can corn, drained
- 1 red pepper, diced
- 1 small red onion, diced
- 1 avocado, diced
- Juice of 1 lime
- 2 tablespoons of olive oil
- Salt and pepper to taste
- Optional: Fresh cilantro, chopped

*Instruction:*

- In a large bowl, combine the black beans, corn, red pepper, red onion and avocado.
- In a small bowl, mix the lime juice, olive oil, salt and pepper.
- Pour the dressing over the salad and toss to combine.
- Garnish with fresh cilantro if desired. Serve immediately or refrigerate for up to 2 days.

## 2. Chicken and vegetable stir-fry

Preparation time: 15 minutes

Cooking time: 10 minutes

Servings: 4

## Ingredients:

- 2 boneless skinless chicken breasts, thinly sliced
- 1 tablespoon of vegetable oil
- 1 large carrot, julienned
- 1 bell pepper, sliced
- 1 cup broccoli florets
- 1 small onion, sliced
- 2 cloves of garlic, minced
- 1/4 cup low-sodium soy sauce
- 2 tablespoons hoisin sauce
- 1 tablespoon of cornstarch mixed with 2 tablespoons of water

## Instruction:

- Heat the vegetable oil in a large skillet or wok over medium-high heat.

- Add chicken and cook until browned and cooked through, about 5-7 minutes. Remove the chicken from the pan and set aside.
- Add carrots, peppers, broccoli and onions to the same pan. Fry for 5 minutes, stirring constantly, until the vegetables are soft.
- Add the garlic and cook for 1 minute more.
- Return the chicken to the pan. Stir in soy sauce, hoisin sauce, and cornstarch mixture. Cook for 2-3 minutes until the sauce thickens.
- Serve immediately, with rice or noodles to taste.

### 3. Vegetable and lentil soup

Preparation time: 10 minutes

Cooking time: 30 minutes

Servings: 6

*Ingredients:*

- 1 tablespoon of olive oil
- 1 onion, diced
- 2 cloves of garlic, minced

- 2 carrots, diced
- 2 stalks of celery, diced
- 1 cup dried lentils, rinsed
- 1 can of diced tomatoes
- 6 cups of vegetable broth
- 1 teaspoon of dried thyme
- 1 bay leaf
- Salt and pepper to taste
- Optional: Fresh parsley, chopped

## *Instruction:*

- Heat the olive oil in a large pot over medium heat. Add the onion and garlic and cook until softened, about 5 minutes.
- Add the carrots and celery and cook for another 5 minutes.
- Stir in the lentils, chopped tomatoes, vegetable stock, thyme and bay leaf.
- Bring to the boil, then reduce the heat and simmer for 25-30 minutes until the lentils are tender.
- Remove the bay leaf and season with salt and pepper to taste.

- Garnish with fresh parsley if desired and serve hot.

## 4. Baked Sweet Potatoes with Black Bean Salsa

Preparation time: 10 minutes

Cooking time: 45 minutes

Servings: 4

### *Ingredients:*

- 4 medium sweet potatoes
- 1 can of black beans, drained and rinsed
- 1 cup corn kernels (fresh, frozen, or canned)
- 1 small red onion, diced
- 1 jalapeno, seeded and minced
- 1/4 cup fresh cilantro, chopped
- Juice of 1 lime
- Salt and pepper to taste

### *Instruction:*

- Preheat oven to 400°F (200°C). Pierce the sweet potatoes with a fork and place them on a baking sheet.

- Bake sweet potatoes for 45 minutes to 1 hour, until tender.
- While the sweet potatoes are baking, prepare the black bean salsa. In a large bowl, combine the black beans, corn, red onion, jalapeno, cilantro, lime juice, salt and pepper.
- Once the sweet potatoes are cooked, let them cool slightly. Cut a slit in the top of each potato and fluff the inside with a fork.
- Top each sweet potato with a generous helping of black bean salsa. Serve immediately.

## 5. Quinoa and peppers stuffed with vegetables

Preparation time: 15 minutes

Cooking time: 30 minutes

Servings: 4

### *Ingredients:*

- 4 peppers, cut off the tops and remove the seeds
- 1 cup quinoa, rinsed
- 2 cups of vegetable broth

- 1 tablespoon of olive oil
- 1 onion, diced
- 2 cloves of garlic, minced
- 1 zucchini, diced
- 1 can of diced tomatoes
- 1 teaspoon of dried oregano
- Salt and pepper to taste
- Optional: Grated cheese for topping

***Instruction:***

- Preheat oven to 375°F (190°C).
- Bring vegetable broth to a boil in a medium saucepan. Add the quinoa, reduce the heat, cover and cook for 15 minutes, until the quinoa is cooked and the stock is absorbed. Fluff with a fork.
- While the quinoa is cooking, heat the olive oil in a large skillet over medium heat. Add the onion and garlic and cook until softened, about 5 minutes.
- Add the zucchini and cook for another 5 minutes.

- Stir in the cooked quinoa, chopped tomatoes, oregano, salt and pepper. Cook for 2-3 minutes until heated through.
- Stuff each pepper with the quinoa and vegetable mixture. Place the stuffed peppers in the baking dish.
- If desired, sprinkle grated cheese over each stuffed pepper.
- Bake in the preheated oven for 20-25 minutes until the peppers soften and the filling is heated through.
- Serve hot.

# CHAPTER 10

## SMOOTHIES AND DRINKS

Smoothies and drinks can be a delicious and nutritious addition to your weight loss journey. They are versatile, quick to prepare and can be full of vitamins, minerals and other nutrients essential for a healthy diet. This chapter will provide you with various recipes for smoothies and drinks that are filling and at the same time low in calories. Each recipe includes step-by-step instructions so you can easily incorporate them into your daily routine.

## 1. Green Detox Smoothie

### *Ingredients:*

- 1 cup spinach
- 1/2 cup cucumber, sliced
- 1/2 green apple, chopped
- 1/2 a banana
- 1 teaspoon of chia seeds
- 1 cup coconut water
- Juice of 1/2 lemon

### *Instruction:*

- Mix: Add all ingredients to a blender.
- Blend until smooth: Blend on high until the mixture is smooth and creamy.
- Serve: Pour into a glass and serve immediately.
- Nutritional information (per serving):

- Calories: 150
- Protein: 3 g
- Carbohydrates: 35 g
- Fat: 2 g

## 2. Berry Protein Smoothie

*Ingredients:*

- 1 cup mixed fruit (strawberries, blueberries, raspberries)
- 1/2 cup plain Greek yogurt
- 1/2 cup almond milk
- 1 spoon of honey
- 1 scoop of vanilla protein powder

*Instruction:*

- Blend: Place all ingredients in a blender.
- Mix: Blend until smooth and creamy.
- Serve: Pour into a glass and enjoy immediately.
- Nutritional information (per serving):
- Calories: 220
- Protein: 20 g
- Carbohydrates: 25 g

- Fat: 4g

## 3. Tropical Paradise Smoothie

*Ingredients:*

- 1/2 cup pineapple chunks
- 1/2 cup mango chunks
- 1/2 a banana
- 1 cup coconut milk
- 1 tablespoon of flax seeds

*Instruction:*

- Mix: Add all ingredients to a blender.
- Mix well: Blend on high until mixture is smooth.
- Serve: Pour into a glass and serve immediately.

*Nutritional information (per serving):*

- Calories: 200
- Protein: 2 g
- Carbohydrates: 45 g
- Fat: 4g

## 4. Spicy citrus green tea

*Ingredients:*

- 1 green tea bag
- 1 cup hot water
- Juice of 1 orange
- Juice of 1/2 lemon
- 1/2 teaspoon ground ginger
- 1/4 teaspoon cayenne pepper
- Honey to taste (optional)

*Instruction:*

- Cooking: Soak a green tea bag in hot water for 3-5 minutes.
- Mix: Add orange juice, lemon juice, ground ginger and cayenne pepper. Mix well.
- Sweetening: Add honey as needed.
- Serve: Enjoy hot or let cool and serve over ice.

*Nutritional information (per serving):*

- Calories: 60
- Protein: 0 g
- Carbohydrates: 15 g
- Fat: 0g

- 5. Avocado spinach smoothie
- Ingredients:
- 1/2 ripe avocado
- 1 cup spinach
- 1/2 a banana
- 1 cup almond milk
- 1 spoon of honey
- 1 teaspoon of chia seeds

*Instruction:*

- Mix: Mix all the ingredients in a blender.
- Blend until smooth: Blend on high until smooth and creamy.
- Serve: Pour into a glass and enjoy immediately.

*Nutritional information (per serving):*

- Calories: 250
- Protein: 4 g
- Carbohydrates: 35 g
- Fat: 12g

**Tips for making the perfect smoothie**

- Use frozen fruit: Provides a thick and creamy texture without the need for ice.
- Balance your ingredients: Aim for a mix of fruits, vegetables, protein and healthy fats to keep you full and full of energy.
- Experiment with liquids: Try different liquids like almond milk, coconut water, or even plain water to find your favorite consistency and flavor.
- Sweeten naturally: Use fruit like bananas, dates or a touch of honey for natural sweetness.
- Add super foods: Fortify your smoothie with super foods like chia seeds, flax seeds or protein powder for added nutrition.

By incorporating these nutritious smoothies and drinks into your diet, you can enjoy delicious flavours while staying on track with your weight loss goals. These recipes are designed to be practical, easy to prepare and packed with essential nutrients to support your journey to a healthier you.

# CONCLUSION

Congratulations on taking a major step toward a healthier and happier you by exploring "Slim and Happy: Great Recipes for Weight Loss." This cookbook was created with the goal of making your weight loss journey enjoyable, sustainable and above all delicious.

On these pages, you've discovered a variety of recipes – from hearty breakfasts to satisfying dinners, quick snacks to refreshing drinks – that prove you don't have to sacrifice taste for health. Each recipe is designed to be practical, easy to follow, and packed with nutrients to support your weight loss goals.

## ADOPTING A HEALTHIER LIFESTYLE

Losing weight isn't just about the numbers on the scale; it's about creating lasting habits that contribute to your overall well-being. By choosing healthy and balanced meals, you give your body the fuel it needs to function optimally. Remember that small, consistent changes lead to significant, lasting results.

## STAY MOTIVATED AND CONSISTENT

The journey to weight loss and better health can be challenging, but also incredibly rewarding. Celebrate your successes, no matter how small, and learn from any setbacks without getting discouraged. Stay consistent, keep trying new recipes, and feel free to modify them to suit your personal tastes and nutritional needs.

## ADDITIONAL RESOURCES

To further support your journey, consider exploring additional resources:

Fitness apps: Track your progress and stay motivated with apps that offer exercise routines and meal planning.

Support groups: Join online communities or local groups to share experiences, tips and encouragement.

Nutritionists and dietitians: Seek expert advice to tailor your diet to your specific needs and goals.

Final thoughts

Your commitment to a healthier lifestyle is commendable. By making informed food choices and enjoying the process of preparing nutritious meals, you are investing in your long-term health and happiness. Remember, this is not just a diet, but a sustainable way of life. Go on a journey, enjoy the flavours and celebrate the positive changes in your life.

For letting "Slim & Satisfy: Delicious Weight Loss Recipes" be a part of your journey. Here's to delicious meals, satisfying results, and a healthier you!

*Thank you.*

Made in the USA
Las Vegas, NV
11 January 2025